Quit Smoking for Good

Your Mind-Body Guide to Beating Nicotine Addiction

Frieda B. May

QUIT SMOKING FOR GOOD

Your Mind–Body Guide to Beating Nicotine Addictio

FRIEDA B. MAY

Copyright Information

Important Note

This book offers a strong, science-backed way to quit smoking for good. By combining mind-body methods with practical tools, it leads and supports you on your journey to freedom from nicotine addiction. However, it's important to know the following:

Success Requires Commitment:

Quitting smoking is a personal journey, and eventually, its success hangs on your dedication and willingness to face challenges. This program equips you with effective strategies and tools, but remember, the choice to quit and beat hurdles rests with you. Be prepared to put in the effort, accept failures as learning opportunities, and never give up on your desire to live a smoke-free life.

Individualized Journeys:

Everyone's quit journey is unique. Some may experience a smooth shift, while others may face setbacks and roadblocks. This is completely normal. Don't get frustrated if you face difficulties. Use every opportunity as a chance to learn and improve your approach. Remember, growth, not perfection, is the key. Embrace the individual nature of your journey and enjoy every step forward.

Visit Your Doctor:

Before starting this program, especially if you have any underlying health conditions, take medications, or are considering using nicotine replacement therapy (NRT), make sure to visit your doctor or other healthcare worker. They

can offer personalized help, ensure your quit plan is safe and appropriate for
you, and provide additional support if needed.

Table Of Contents

Overview

Nicotine addiction is a complicated fight, fought on both physical and mental fronts. Traditional quit-smoking methods often fail because they overemphasize grit and ignore the psychological traps that keep you hooked.

Quit Smoking for Good: Your Mind-Body Guide to Beating Nicotine Addiction empowers you to break free with a new method that blends science-backed techniques, useful tools, and compassionate support.

This book leads you through every stage of your journey:

- **Understanding Your Enemy:** Discover the science behind nicotine's hold on your brain and how it hijacks your reward systems. Identify your personal smoke cues and trends.

- **Prepare for Freedom:** Create a clear quit plan, tap into your deep-seated drive, and create a strong support system.

- **Your Quitting Toolkit:** Master deep breathing techniques to fight cravings, develop awareness to handle stress, and learn how to retrain your brain's reward pathways.

- **The First Days:** Navigate the expected physical and mental hurdles with proven tactics, and celebrate every milestone to reinforce your progress.
- **Your Smoke-Free Life:** Rebuild healthy habits, find joy in everyday activities, and explore new ways to treat yourself. Learn to expect slip-ups and build resilience for ongoing success.

Unlike other tools, this book goes beyond simply telling you to stop smoking. It allows you to:

- Outsmart nicotine's brain tricks
- Manage urges effectively with mind-body tools
- Find real pleasure in a smoke-free life
- Build a support system that truly helps
- Stay quit, not just for a few days or weeks, but forever

If you're ready for a lasting answer, Quit Smoking for Good is your plan for reclaiming your freedom, health, and the satisfying life you deserve.

Introduction: Breaking Free

Imagine, for a moment, a life without the steady cloud of cigarettes. No more sneaking looks at the clock, counting the minutes until your next break. No more stale smell sticking to your clothes, the critical glances, or the nagging worry etched into your loved ones' eyes. Picture yourself energetic, focused, and finally in full control. This is the promise of freedom from smoking addiction, and it's within your reach.

You've probably tried to quit before. Perhaps you fought through willpower alone, gritting your teeth through terrible withdrawals. Maybe you tried patches, gum, or even those strange e-cigarettes, only to find yourself right back where you started. The truth is, most standard quit-smoking ways fail, and it's not your fault. They often focus solely on the physical nicotine addiction, ignoring the strong mental and emotional chains that keep you hooked.

Why Nicotine Wins

Nicotine is a clever foe. It infiltrates your brain, stealing your normal reward system. Every puff supports the idea that cigarettes bring relief, joy, or focus. Soon, your brain starts associating smoking with nearly everything you do – your morning coffee, stressful work calls, and times of joy. These links become so deeply ingrained that trying to quit feels like breaking up with a demanding, controlling partner.

The urges are persistent. The withdrawal pangs through your body make it difficult to think about anything besides lighting up. But here's the secret that the nicotine business doesn't want you to know: much of the pain involved with quitting is manufactured by your own mind.

The Missing Piece

That's where this book comes in. Unlike other quit-smoking books that treat you like a bundle of grit waiting to be activated, we're going to change the script. We'll dig into the science behind addiction, revealing nicotine's tricks so you can outsmart them. But the game-changer lies in controlling the amazing power of your mind and body.

Think of your body as a clever machine, always trying for balance. You have built-in methods for managing worry and discomfort. Nicotine has merely put a brief block on them. With the right tools, including easy deep breathing techniques, you can begin to recover that natural balance, making cravings less intense.

At the same time, we'll work on rewiring your brain. You'll learn to spot the mental traps that lead to smoking and replace them with healthier thinking habits. It's about breaking old connections and building new, powerful ones. This isn't about gritting your teeth and surviving – it's about finding real freedom.

A Journey, Not a Miracle

Let's be clear: stopping smoking isn't magic. It takes dedication and a readiness to face some initial discomfort. But it won't be the constant pain you might expect. With each passing day, you'll gain more power. The cravings will fade, your energy will return, and you'll rediscover a sense of pride and success that no cigarette could ever give.

This book is your guide on this journey. We'll provide step-by-step methods, science-backed insights, and lots of unwavering support. It's time to break nicotine's hold on your life and step into the freedom you deserve.

This is your moment. Let's begin.

Chapter 1: Know Your Enemy

Nicotine's Impact on the Brain: The Science of Addiction

To beat nicotine, you need to understand its methods. Let's pull back the curtain and reveal the science behind how this seemingly simple substance infiltrates your brain and creates the strong grip of addiction.

The Hijacked Reward System

Your brain is wired with a complex reward system intended to reinforce actions important for life. Every time you eat great food, enjoy a laugh with friends or experience a sense of success, your brain releases a surge of dopamine – a feel-good chemical that signals, "This is important! Do it again!"

Nicotine cruelly hijacks this normal system. It mimics a neurotransmitter called acetylcholine, which plays a role in motivation, attention, and learning. When you inhale cigarette smoke, nicotine floods your brain, causing a huge, unnatural release of dopamine. Your brain misinterprets this manufactured rise as a signal that smoking is awesome and important to your well-being.

The Illusion of Relief

With continued smoking, your brain adjusts to this constant nicotine attack. It starts to turn down its own dopamine production and lowers the number of available dopamine receptors. Now, even normal tasks don't feel as satisfying as they used to.

What happens when nicotine levels start to drop between cigarettes? You begin to experience withdrawal symptoms: irritability, anxiety, and difficulty focusing. It's not just your body wanting a physical drug; your brain is desperate for that dopamine hit to feel "normal" again. Smoking brings false comfort, continuing a never-ending loop of craving and reward.

The Mental Trap

It's important to remember that physical addiction is only part of the issue. As nicotine reshapes your brain chemistry, it also forges strong mental connections. Your brain learns to link smoking with nearly everything:

- **Stressful situations:** The illusion of nicotine calming your nerves encourages the belief that a cigarette is the answer.

- **Social settings:** Rituals like smoking breaks with peers or an after-dinner cigarette hardwire social link to nicotine.
- **Emotions:** Boredom, anger, and even happiness, can all become causes for lighting up.

These associations become so automatic that merely the sight of a pack of cigarettes, smelling smoke, or even just having a few minutes to yourself can trigger strong cravings.

The Three Components of Addiction

True obsession can be understood in three parts:

1. **Physical Dependence:** Your body gets accustomed to a steady amount of nicotine. Withdrawal happens when it doesn't have it.
2. **Tolerance:** Over time, the same amount of nicotine causes a less satisfying dopamine hit, making you crave more.
3. **Psychological Dependence:** The mental and emotional idea that you need nicotine to function, cope with life and feel pleasure.

Traditional stopping ways often focus solely on physical dependence, leaving you to fight the psychological parts on your own. This is a recipe for return.

Cravings: Not Just Physical

Withdrawal signs, those terrible feelings when you try to quit, are both physical and psychological. Physically, your body misses the tobacco it's become hooked on. But mentally, your brain fights too. It's used to smoking linked with certain actions and feelings:

- **The Morning Ritual:** The first smoke with coffee sets a pattern for the day.
- **Stress Buster:** Smoking is misunderstood as a way to calm down when it feeds anxiety long-term.
- **Boredom** Breaker: Lighting up becomes a backup when you lack better ways to excite yourself.
- **Social Crutch:** Smoking is often linked to mingling, making it tough to stop without feeling isolated.

The Good News: Your Brain Can Heal

The human brain is incredibly flexible. While nicotine causes permanent changes, it is definitely possible to retrain your brain, break those connections, and recover a healthier reward system. The first days and weeks might involve some pain, but as nicotine's hold weakens, you'll find amazing resilience.

Think about it this way: You aren't giving up cigarettes; you're getting back your brain's natural ability to find joy, handle stress, and experience life on its own terms. Understanding the facts is your first tool. Awareness helps you to outsmart those constant urges and see them for what they are: a brief trick of a chemically altered brain, not a true need.

Knowledge is Power

Understanding how nicotine works on your brain does a few important things:

1. **Disrupts the Illusion:** You're no longer just a 'bad smoker' who lacks willpower. You're fighting modified brain chemistry.

2. **Reduces Fear:** Withdrawal is temporary. Knowing your brain will heal makes it less scary.

3. **Boosts Motivation:** With every day smoke-free, you're regaining your brain's natural balance and control.

Let's move on to discovering your personal smoking story, helping you spot the unique triggers and patterns that have kept you entangled with nicotine.

Your Smoking Story: Identifying Triggers and Habits

To beat an enemy, you must first understand their methods. This is especially true when it comes to smoking abuse. Before we dive into the strategies for breaking its hold on you, it's important to get a clear picture of your unique smoking story. This chapter is all about self-awareness—the key to breaking free from those mindless habits that keep you reaching for a cigarette.

The Smoking Journal

Your first task is to become a detective. Grab a notebook or use a note-taking app on your phone. For the next few days, your goal is to track each time you smoke and jot down these details:

- **Time and Date:** When do you light up? First thing in the morning? Midday breaks? After meals?

- **Craving Level:** Rate the strength of your urge to smoke on a range of 1 to 5 (5 being an almost unbearable need).
- **Situation:** What are you doing right before you smoke? Working? Driving? Socializing? Relaxing?
- **Location:** Where are you when the urge strikes? At home? In the car? At your desk?
- **Feelings:** How are you feeling emotionally? Stressed? Bored? Happy? Anxious?
- **Company:** Are you alone or with others? Are specific people triggers for you?

Don't judge yourself during this process. This isn't about guilt or shame; it's about gathering knowledge with the interest of a scientist.

Analyzing Your Data

After several days of tracking, it's time to look for trends. Ask yourself:

- **When do my greatest cravings hit?** Do certain times of day bring more of a challenge?
- **What situations regularly lead to smoking?** Are work breaks, stressful phone calls, or specific social events your biggest triggers?

- **Are my urges tied to emotions?** Do you smoke to handle worry, boredom, or other difficult feelings?
- **Are there regular places where I light up?** Does your home surroundings or car spark the urge?
- **Do certain people affect my smoking?** Do you tend to smoke more with specific friends or colleagues?

Trigger Categories

Your causes likely fall into several categories:

- **Situational Triggers:** Activities or places that you strongly link with smoking (coffee breaks, driving, the end of a meal)
- **Emotional Triggers:** Feelings that drive you to seek the imagined comfort of a cigarette (stress, boredom, worry)
- **Social Triggers:** Specific people or social settings that increase the urge to smoke
- **Withdrawal Triggers:** Symptoms of nicotine withdrawal (restlessness, anger) that can trick you into reaching for another smoke.

The Power of Awareness

Simply noticing these causes is an incredibly powerful first step. When you're aware that ending a work job might lead to a craving, you're not caught off guard. You can prepare a dealing plan in advance. If you know mingling with a specific friend makes you want to smoke, you can make an informed choice about whether to see them early in your quitting journey. Awareness gives you back a feeling of power.

Triggers Aren't Forever

It's important to remember that your triggers won't always hold the same power over you. As you break your addiction, the association between a setting (like your morning coffee) and the desire to smoke will gradually lessen. However, in those early days of quitting take extra care.

Your personalized battle plan

As we move through the book, we'll create specific techniques for dealing with each type of trigger. The self-knowledge you've gained in this chapter is like making your own personal map of the enemy's area. You'll know where the dangers lie and be able to strategically make your way around them.

A Note on Cravings

Cravings are a normal part of beating nicotine addiction. Nicotine has briefly short-circuited your brain's reward system, and it takes time to reset. Understanding your triggers helps you anticipate these cravings, and as you learn the coping strategies in the following chapters, those urges will become increasingly doable.

Ready to move forward? The next part is all about getting ready for your final battle with nicotine!

Chapter 2: Prepare for Freedom

Setting Your Quit Date: Strategies for Success

Picture this: a distinct line in the sand, a marker on your calendar, a day that represents a turning point. Your cease date is more than just a number; it's a declaration of your intention to change and a potent tool for getting ready to quit. Choosing the right date can significantly influence your success, so let's delve into the best strategies for making that decision.

The Right Time: Is it Now or Later?

- **The Cold Turkey Approach:** For some, immediate action feels empowering. If you have a strong sense of resolve and a supportive environment, ceasing cold turkey can work. The benefits? You rip off the bandage swiftly and initiate the withdrawal process.
- **The Gradual Reduction:** If the notion of going from an inveterate smoker to a non-smoker overnight feels burdensome, tapering your nicotine consumption over a few weeks can ease the

transition. Set small, achievable reduction objectives to progressively lessen your dependence.

- **The Target Date:** Setting a date a little distance in the future (2-4 weeks) is the most prevalent approach for a good reason. It grants you time to:

1. **Mentally Prepare:** Visualize your smoke-free existence, develop your motivation, and anticipate challenges.

2. **Gather Support:** Alert friends and family, enlist aid (counseling, support groups, etc.), and ask for their forbearance and encouragement.

3. **Practical Steps:** Ditch lighters, ashtrays, and any remaining cigarettes. Stock up on healthful alternatives like straws, gum, or crunchy treats.

Factors to Consider When Choosing Your Quit Date:

- **Stress Levels:** Pick a time comparatively free of significant upheavals or unavoidable stressors (if possible). Quitting can be distressing in itself, so minimize external pressures.

- **Triggers:** If certain events, locations, or people are significant smoking triggers, consider selecting a period where those can be avoided or managed.

- **Symbolic Significance:** Choosing a meaningful date like a birthday, anniversary, or even the Great American Smokeout (third Thursday of November) can lend extra motivation.

- **Don't Overthink It:** While a bit of planning is wise, don't let the quest for the "perfect day" be an excuse to delay. Sometimes, the finest day is the day you determine enough is enough.

The Quit Date Countdown: Your Preparation Checklist

Once your date is determined, use the time wisely to position yourself up for success:

- **Track Your Smoking Habits:** For a few days, log every time you smoke. Note not just the cigarette, but your demeanor, location, and what you're doing. This develops awareness of your triggers.

- **Practice Coping Skills:** Start experimenting with deep breathing or other relaxation techniques. These will be your lifelines during desires.

- **Line Up Your Support:** Communicate honestly with loved ones and get their commitment to assisting you through the process.
- **Identify Your "Whys":** Create a potent list of reasons for resigning. Focus on the positive – enhanced health, financial freedom, establishing a good example. Carry this list with you and look at it frequently.

A Note on Slip-Ups

If you discover yourself smoking before your cessation date, don't use it as an excuse to give up! Analyze what transpired, learn from it, and recommit to your end date as if nothing changed. Every endeavor, even an imperfect one, advances you closer to success.

Your Quit Date Is a Promise

Circle your cessation date on the calendar with a vibrant, bold marker. It's a covenant to yourself, a commitment to taking control. From this day forward, you are actively striving toward a healthier, smoke-free future.

Finding Your Why: Reclaiming Your Motivation

Wanting to resign and genuinely being ready to cease are two distinct things. Before embarking on this voyage, it's crucial to reconnect with the deep-rooted reasons that fuel your desire for liberation. This 'why' will be your anchor during difficult moments, reminding you of the greater goal when cravings attempt to draw you back.

- **The Cost of Smoking:** Go beyond generic health concerns. Get specific. Calculate how much money you spend on cigarettes each week, month, and year. Think about what else you could do with that money. Are there experiences you're losing out on, a healthier lifestyle you could afford, or loved ones you could treat?

- **Your Health Ledger:** Make a list of how smoking has already impacted your body. Do you get fatigued easily? Have recurrent coughs? Notice alterations to your skin? Now, visualize yourself smoke-free. Imagine increased vitality, enhanced breathing, and a more youthful appearance.

- **Beyond Yourself:** Think about the individuals in your life who are affected by your smoking. How does concern about your well-being impact them? Are there loved ones who urgently want you to quit? Picture their delight and relief when you succeed.

- **The Freedom List:** Envision your optimal smoke-free day. What would you do with the extra time? Would you rise up earlier for a revitalizing walk? Spend more quality time with your family. Imagine the sense of accomplishment without the incessant interruptions of cigarette breaks.

Exercise: Your 'Why' Statement

Take some time to reflect on your responses to the queries above. Now, compose a compelling, personalized 'why' statement. Here are some examples:

- "I'm stopping for my health, so I can have the energy to play with my grandchildren without breathing for air."
- "I'm quitting to reclaim my freedom, save money, and finally take that dream vacation."
- "I'm stopping to show my children that I choose them over any drug."

Write your statement down and position it somewhere visible. Read it daily, letting it fuel your determination.

Building Your Support System: You're Not Alone

Quitting smoking is challenging, but it doesn't have to be a lonely endeavor. Surrounding yourself with a robust support network is one of the greatest predictors of success. Here's how to construct your ideal team:

- **Identify Your Champions:** Think about the individuals in your life who are authentically supportive of your decision to quit. This could be your companion, family members, close acquaintances, or even a trusted healthcare professional.

- **Communicate Your Needs:** Be honest about how your loved ones can assist. Do you need someone to listen when cravings strike, distract you with enjoyable activities, or simply offer non-judgmental encouragement?

- **Online Communities:** Tap into the tremendous power of online support groups and forums dedicated to abandoning smoking. Connect with others going through the same voyage, share experiences, and celebrate victories together.

- **Professional Help:** If you've struggled to cease in the past or have additional health concerns, don't hesitate to seek professional guidance. Therapists specializing in addiction and smoking cessation programs can provide tailored support.

- **Quitting Buddies:** If you know someone else who's attempting to cease, consider teaming up. Hold each other accountable, share ideas, and encourage each other during challenging moments.

Important: Setting Boundaries

It's acceptable and even necessary to set boundaries with those who may not initially support your decision. Kindly but firmly request that they don't smoke around you or offer you cigarettes. If someone's negativity becomes too disruptive, consider limiting your time with them temporarily. ***Your journey to liberation deserves to be protected.***

Exercise 1: The "Why" Collage

- **Purpose**: To visually reinforce your reasons for resigning, making your "why" tangible and impactful.
- **Materials:** Magazines, scissors, adhesive, poster board or large paper.

Instructions:

1. Flip through magazines, searching for images and words that resonate with your motivations for quitting. These could be pictures of healthful activities, happy families, travel destinations, financial objectives, or anything related to your personal motivations.

2. Cut out the images and text, arranging them on the poster board.

3. Feel free to add your own writing, illustrations, or embellishments that further personalize the collage.

4. Display your collage conspicuously where you'll see it every day as a reminder of your commitment.

Exercise 2: Letter to Your Future Self

- Purpose: To bridge the divide between your current resolve and the potential challenges that may arise, solidifying your dedication.

- Materials: Pen and paper, or your preferred digital notetaking instrument.

Instructions:

1. Imagine yourself one year from now, having successfully stopped for good.

2. Write a letter to that future expressing gratitude for making this life-changing decision.

3. Describe how your smoke-free life has improved – increased vitality, greater health, financial savings, stronger relationships.

4. Acknowledge any challenges you overcame and the strategies that helped you remain on track.

5. End with words of encouragement and pride, reminding your future self of the fortitude it took to reach this point.

Exercise 3: Support Network Map

- Purpose: To visually depict your support system and identify any potential gaps
- Materials: Large paper or whiteboard, colorful markers.

Instructions:

1. Draw a large circle in the center, writing "ME" inside.

2. Around the center circle, draw smaller circles representing each person in your support network (family, colleagues, therapist, online communities).

3. Use different colored markers to designate the specific type of support each person or resource offers (listening ear, distraction, accountability, etc.)

4. Analyze your map: Are there certain forms of support that are stronger than others? Are there any locations where you could benefit from additional resources?

Tips for Incorporating Exercises:

- Timing Matters: Suggest doing these exercises early in your cessation journey to reinforce motivation from the very start.

- Revisit and Revise: Encourage readers to return to their collage, letter, and map periodically during their cease voyage. They can add new elements, update their support network, or simply re-read them for a boost of determination.

Remember, you are not a burden by requesting assistance. Your loved ones want to see you succeed, and a strong support system will make all the difference.

Chapter 3: Your Quitting Toolkit

Nicotine cessation can be a roller coaster. Beyond the physical cravings, you'll likely encounter moments of acute tension, restlessness, and anxiety. Your quitting toolkit is all about developing simple yet potent strategies to navigate those surges and emerge stronger.

Mastering Deep Breathing: Your Anytime Craving Buster

Deep breathing isn't just about relaxation – it's about rewiring your body's stress response. Nicotine has trained your body to associate tension with a cigarette. Deep breathing combats this by:

- **Calming the Nervous System:** Deep, leisurely breaths activate the parasympathetic nervous system, responsible for the "rest and digest" response. This counters the fight-or-flight sensations provoked by tension and cravings.
- **Oxygen Boost:** Deep breathing floods your body with oxygen, reducing sensations of tension and enhancing focus. It's your internal refresh switch.

- **Mimicking Smoking Rituals:** The act of slow, intentional inhales and exhales can partially satiate the habitual motions associated with smoking, facilitating the transition.

The Basics of Deep Breathing

- **Find a comfortable, peaceful spot.** You can recline or lie down, whatever feels best.
- **Close your eyes (optional).** This helps focus inward.
- **One hand on the abdomen, one on the pectoral.** This helps you monitor your respiration.
- **Inhale through your nostrils.** Aim to fill your abdomen with oxygen, keeping your thorax mostly still.
- **Pause momentarily.** Hold your breath for a count of 1 or 2 if comfortable.
- **Exhale steadily through your nostrils.** Let your abdomen decompress naturally.
- **Repeat for 5-10 minutes.** Focus solely on the sensation of your respiration.

Practice Makes Perfect

Start practicing deep breathing several times a day, even when you're not yearning for a cigarette. This develops muscle memory, making it a more effective weapon against appetites.

Deep Breathing in the Heat of a Craving

When a craving strikes, your instinct will be to despair. Take a stand:

- **Acknowledge the Craving:** Don't attempt to ignore it. Simply state to yourself, "I'm having a craving, and it's temporary."
- **Start your steady inhaling.** Close your eyes and focus entirely on the sensations of your respiration.
- **Ride the Wave:** Picture the craving like a wave. It will crest and then naturally subside. Breathe through it.

Mindfulness in Action: Managing Stress and Urges

Mindfulness is the discipline of being completely present in the current moment, without judgment. It's a superpower when ceasing smoking because it enables you to:

- **See Your Thoughts Clearly:** Mindfulness helps you observe your cravings and the thoughts that sustain them ("I need this," "I can't handle this"). This separation creates space between you and the urge.

- **Manage Stress Proactively:** Mindfulness allows you to capture stress early on before it escalates into a craving. You can then deploy tools like deep breathing to regain control.

- **Replace Autopilot:** Smoking is often an unconscious habit. Mindfulness trains you to be more aware of your triggers, choices, and actions.

Simple Mindfulness Exercises

- **Body Scan:** Sit comfortably and apply your attention to each part of your body, from toes to cranium. Notice sensations of warmth, quivering, and tension – simply observe, without attempting to change anything.

- **Mindful Eating:** Choose a modest snack like a slice of fruit. Engage all your senses – gaze at its textures, inhale its aroma, and savor each bite slowly.

-
- **Walking Meditation:** Focus entirely on the sensations of each step – your feet connecting with the ground, your body moving through space.

Mindfulness is a skill that strengthens with practice. The more you cultivate mindfulness in ordinary life, the greater the weapon it becomes against cravings and tension.

The Power of Distraction: Shifting Your Focus

Sometimes, pure willpower and breathing techniques won't wholly make a craving disappear. That's where strategic distraction comes into play. The aim is to interrupt the mental loop of craving by diverting your attention to a different activity. Here's how:

- **Your Distraction Arsenal:** Prepare a go-to list of engaging activities that work for you. They should be readily accessible and provide a healthy dose of distraction. Some ideas:

1. **Physical activity:** A brisk walk, brief exercise, or even a few jumping jacks.
2. **Creativity:** Drawing, playing a musical instrument, or writing in a journal.

3. **Mind Games:** Puzzles, Sudoku, or a challenging mobile game.

4. **Something Soothing:** Taking a hot shower, listening to tranquil music, or spending time with a companion.

- **The 10-Minute Rule:** When a craving strikes hard, commit to engaging in your selected distraction for just 10 minutes. Often, the pinnacle of the craving will pass by the time you're done, and you'll have spared yourself from lighting up.

- **Change Your Environment:** If practicable, get up and move to a new location. Go outside, and visit a different room – this change of scenery can help disrupt the yearning cycle.

- **The Power of Small Tasks:** Break down a daunting craving into a succession of micro-tasks. Instead of "I have to get through this," think: "I just need to put on my shoes, then open the door, then walk for 2 minutes..." It makes the hurdle seem more manageable.

If You Slip Up: Relapse Prevention and Compassion

Quitting smoking is rarely a direct line. Slip-ups can happen, particularly in the early days. The most essential issue is how you respond to the slip-up. Beating yourself up will only undermine your efforts. Instead, approach it with these principles:

- **Compassion is Key:** You're combating a potent addiction, and setbacks are part of the process. Instead of self-condemnation, offer yourself the same compassion you would a friend.

- **Analyze, Don't Catastrophize:** Examine what triggered the slip-up. Was it tension, a particular situation, or exposure to a smoking cue? Identifying the cause helps you plan to avoid it in the future.

- **It's a Slip-up, Not a Failure:** One cigarette doesn't negate all your progress. Don't fall into the trap of "I've already blown it, might as well finish the pack."

- **Get Back on Track ASAP:** Don't let the slip-up become an excuse to give up utterly. Revisit your 'why', practice deep breathing, and recommit to your cessation journey. Each moment is a new start.

- **Reach Out:** If you're struggling, don't hesitate to rely on your support system. A motivational talk or a venting session with a trusted individual can make all the difference.

Recall that giving up smoking is a journey, not a quick fix. Treat setbacks as opportunities to learn, strengthen your resolve, and build even greater resilience for the road ahead.

Chapter 4: The First Days: What to Expect

The first few days after stopping smoking are often the most difficult. Your body is changing to being nicotine-free, and withdrawal signs can kick in. Understanding what to expect is key to getting through this brief pain and into the better days ahead.

Common Withdrawal Symptoms

Everyone experiences withdrawal slightly differently, but here are some typical ones to be aware of:

- **Cravings:** These will be strong at first, especially in scenarios you associate with smoking. Each desire will last only a few minutes, but they can feel persistent. Your deep breathing and other tools will be lifelines.
- **Irritability, Anger, or Restlessness:** It's normal to feel on edge as your brain re-adjusts. Be gentle with yourself and others as these feelings pass.

- **Difficulty Concentrating:** "Brain fog" can be annoying but is brief. Take breaks, do small bursts of focused work, and avoid juggling when possible.
- **Sleep Disturbances:** Vivid thoughts and trouble going or staying asleep are usual. A regular sleep routine can help.
- **Increased Appetite:** You may be tempted to replace smoke with food. Opt for healthy food, and plenty of water, and keep amounts reasonable.

The Timeline of Withdrawal

- **First 24-72 Hours:** Symptoms usually peak during this time. Hang in there, it gets better!
- **One Week:** Most acute physical complaints will begin to lessen. Mentally, you may still have ups and downs.
- **Two Weeks:** You're through the worst! Cravings lessen, and your energy and attention start to improve.
- **One Month & Beyond:** Continue to be cautious, but day by day, you'll build greater resilience and trust in your smoke-free life.

Managing Discomfort: Your Toolkit

- **Deep Breathing & Mindfulness:** Your go-to tools against cravings and worry.

- **Hydration:** Drink plenty of water. Nicotine detox can be dehydrating.

- **Healthy Movement:** Exercise is a natural mood-booster and worry relief. Even short walks help.

- **Distraction:** Plan activities to keep your thoughts busy – games, puzzles, a new hobby.

- **Rest:** Allow yourself extra sleep if needed. Your body is working hard to readjust.

- **Treat Yourself:** Reward your progress with small pleasures unrelated to smoking.

Important Notes

- **Talk to Your Doctor:** If your withdrawal symptoms are serious, there may be medical choices to provide relief.

- **Nicotine Replacement Therapy (NRT):** If suggested by your doctor, NRT (patches, gum, etc.) can ease the change. Remember, the goal is to be nicotine-free totally.

This is Temporary

Repeat this like a prayer! Withdrawal sensations are a sign your body is healing. They may be uncomfortable, but they won't last forever. Remind yourself of your 'why', lean on your support system, and enjoy every hour and day of greater freedom.

Emotional Rollercoaster: Strategies for Staying Balanced

The first few days of stopping are often a whirlwind of feelings. Elation and pride mix with anger, nervousness, and even sadness. It's your brain and body recalibrating. Prepare yourself, and have tactics ready:

- **Expect the Mood Swings:** Knowing that mood changes are normal lessens their power. Remind yourself, "This is withdrawal, not who I truly am."
- **Self-care is King:** Prioritize good sleep, healthy food, gentle movement, and things that bring you joy or rest. Treat yourself with extra care.
- **Feel Your Feelings:** Avoid bottling up feelings, but don't over-analyze them either. Journaling, talking to a trusted friend, or simply taking a good cry can provide a healthy release.

- **Temporary Distractions:** When intense feelings hit, change your attention. Engage in a simple sport, watch a funny show, or listen to upbeat music.
- **The Low Doesn't Last:** Remind yourself that the mental rollercoaster won't go on forever. Each day brings you closer to greater security.

Celebrating Milestones: Recognizing Your Progress

Quitting smoking is an incredible journey marked by big and small wins. Celebrating your wins keeps you encouraged and reinforces your choice. Here's how:

- **The First Hour, The First Day:** These are huge feats. Acknowledge them and treat yourself with something non-cigarette related (a favorite tea, a relaxed bath, a call with a supporting friend).
- **Track Your Progress:** Use a quitting app, a calendar, or a simple jar where you put the money you save by not buying smokes. Visualizing your success is strong.
- **The One Week Mark:** This is a big milestone! Treat yourself to something special – a massage, a

small gift you've wanted, or an experience rather than an actual item.

- **Ritualize Your Wins:** Mark each milestone with a unique, healthy practice. It could be a special walk in nature, writing in a gratitude book, or enjoying a favorite treat in a mindful way.
- **Don't Compare Your Journey:** Progress isn't straight, and everyone's schedule is different. Celebrate your accomplishments, regardless of what others do.

Bonus: "Future You" Letters

Write yourself several letters from your future smoke-free self. Open one at different stages (one week, one month, six months). Describe how happy you are, how much better you feel, and everything you've gained. It's a beautiful reflection of how far you've come.

Key Takeaway

The early days are about weathering the storm, but don't forget to recognize your amazing strength. Celebrating those goals fuels your energy for the road ahead.

Healthy Reward Ideas

The goal is to develop new, positive memories that replace the short-term benefit formerly given by cigarettes. Choose choices that are truly enjoyable to you:

Experiences over Things:

- A mini-trip to a nearby site
- Tickets to a show, play, or sports event
- A class to learn a new skill (cooking, drawing, dance, etc.)
- A refreshing spa treatment or massage

Boosting Well-Being:

- A lesson with a personal trainer or a fun exercise class
- Upgrading your health practice or getting a facial
- New workout clothes or tools to support healthy habits
- Plants, flowers, or supplies to make a relaxing place

Small Luxuries

- A special coffee or tea you wouldn't usually indulge in Fancy bath products for a relaxing soak
- A new book, podcast, or membership to your favorite magazine
- A warm blanket, beautiful candle, or aromatherapy spray

Acts of Kindness

- Donate the saved money to a cause you believe in
- Treat a close one to a coffee or lunch
- Volunteer your time to help those in need

"Future You" Letters: Structuring for Impact

- Timing is Key: Consider these milestones: 24 hours, 72 hours, 1 week, 2 weeks, 1 month, 3 months, 6 months, 1 year.

Specificity:

- Instead of "I feel better," write, "I can walk up three flights of stairs without getting winded!"
- Paint a picture: "I cooked a delicious dinner and enjoyed it without a single smoke break, and the food tasted amazing!"

Focus on Gains:

- "I've saved \$___, and I'm starting to plan that special trip."
- "My relationships feel stronger because I'm more present and less irritable."
- "I discovered a newfound love for hiking, and my body feels capable."

Words of Encouragement:

- Remind your past self how strong and motivated they are.
- Acknowledge that it might be tough, but stress, "You are doing this, and I'm so proud of you!"
- End each letter with "You won't regret it, I promise."

Additional Tips:

- **Handwritten is Best:** The work makes it extra special.
- **Date Them Clearly:** Put the date you wrote it, not the date you plan to open it.

- **Store Them Strategically:** Place them somewhere you'll come across them, not hidden away to be forgotten.

Chapter 5: Your Smoke-Free Life

You've overcome the hardest part – breaking free from nicotine's grip. Now, it's time to build a lively, satisfying life where cigarettes no longer have a place. This is where healthy habits become your secret tool for keeping your freedom long-term.

Rebuilding Healthy Habits: Nutrition, Exercise, and Self-Care

Nutrition: Fuel Your Transformation

- **Smoking dampens your taste buds. Rediscover the joy of real food**: Focus on whole fruits, veggies, and lean protein sources.

- **Manage cravings wisely:** Keep healthy snacks like nuts, cut-up veggies, or yogurt on hand.

- **Hydration is key:** Drink plenty of water to flush out toxins and ease withdrawal symptoms.

- **Be patient:** Your hunger and digestion will take time to adjust. Avoid extreme diets or limiting yourself too hard.

Exercise: Reclaim Your Energy

- **Start slow:** Even short walks make a difference. Increase exercise gradually as you feel better.
- **Find what you enjoy:** Don't fear exercise! Explore dancing, yoga, swimming, or team sports.
- **Boost your mood:** Exercise is a natural mood enhancer, fighting leftover withdrawal blues.
- **Fitness as a reward:** Use the money you save from not smoking to invest in new workout gear, a gym ticket, or an activity class.

Self-Care: Nurture Your Well-Being

- **Sleep is essential:** Nicotine changes sleep habits. Aim for 7-8 hours of quality sleep for better happiness and energy levels.
- **Manage stress proactively:** Use the deep breathing and focus tools you've learned. Explore stress-reducing activities like yoga, spending time in nature, or artistic skills.
- **Reconnect with joy:** What activities used to bring you the pleasure that smoking may have pushed aside? Rediscover those interests.

- **Forgive slip-ups:** If you do slip up with a cigarette, don't let it grow into a full return. Practice self-compassion, learn from the experience, and return to your goals.

Beyond the Basics

- **Oral Fixation Fix:** Many ex-smokers miss the feeling of having something in their mouths. Try sugar-free gum, crunchy snacks like carrots, herbal teas, or even just holding a pen or straw.
- **Boredom Busters:** Identify scenarios where you used to smoke and build new, healthy habits for those times. Instead of a coffee and smoke break, it may become a quick walk and tea time.
- **Reward Yourself Regularly:** Celebrate non-smoking accomplishments with events and things that support your new healthy lifestyle.

Important Note: It takes time to create new habits. Be patient with yourself, enjoy small wins, and don't hesitate to seek help from a healthcare worker or nutritionist if required.

The Takeaway

Rebuilding a healthy lifestyle isn't about hardship; it's about accepting all that life has to offer when you are no longer ruled by cigarettes. These choices will strengthen your freedom, making a return to smoking less and less attractive with each passing day.

Rewiring Your Reward System: Finding New Pleasures

One of the reasons why stopping smoking can be so hard is that cigarettes have changed your brain's reward system. Every time you light up, you get a surge of dopamine, a chemical that makes you feel good. Over time, your brain learns to associate smoking with happiness and wants more of it.

But the good news is that your brain is incredibly flexible. It can change and rewire itself in reaction to new events. This is called neuroplasticity. When you quit smoking, you give your brain a chance to weaken those dopamine pathways linked to cigarettes and make space for new, healthy links to form.

In this section, we will explore how you can rewire your reward system by finding new joys in life. You will discover a wide range of activities that can stimulate your brain, improve your happiness, and enrich your well-being. You will also learn how to practice awareness, a skill that can help you enjoy any moment, big or small.

Expanding Your Pleasure Horizons

One of the best ways to change your reward system is to try new things. When you subject yourself to new and challenging situations, you activate your brain's curiosity and learning circuits, which release dopamine and other feel-good chemicals. You also increase your sense of self, your skills, and your hobbies.

There are countless things that you can try, based on your preferences, availability, and budget. Here are some examples, grouped into four categories:

1. **Creative:** Learning a new skill (instrument, drawing, writing)

2. **Physical:** Trying different types of exercise (yoga, hiking, swimming)

3. **Social:** Joining a club, helping, taking a group class

4. **Experiential:** Visiting a museum, watching a show, discovering a new part of town

You don't have to limit yourself to one area. You can mix and match, or build your own. The key is to find something that sparks your interest, engages your attention, and tests your skills.

The 30-Day Experiment

To help you find new joys, we challenge you to try one new thing each day for a month. This is not a rigid or stressful task, but a fun and exciting exercise. You can choose any action that appeals to you, as long as it is different from your usual practice.

You can use the examples above as a starting point, or come up with your own ideas. You can also repeat an activity if you loved it, but try to change it slightly (for example, if you played the guitar one day, try a different song or genre the next day).

The goal of this experiment is to subject yourself to a range of stimuli and see what connects with you. You might be shocked by what activities bring you unexpected joy or show hidden talents. You might also discover new parts of yourself or new relationships with others.

To make the most of this project, we suggest that you keep a journal of your encounters. Jot down your actions, feelings, and lessons gained. This will help you reflect on your progress, and select what tasks you want to explore further.

Mindfulness in Action

Another way to change your reward system is to practice awareness. Mindfulness is the ability to focus on the present moment without judgment or distraction. When you are mindful, you are fully aware of your thoughts, feelings, emotions, and surroundings.

Mindfulness can increase the pleasure of any action, big or small. By being aware, you can enjoy the details, nuances, and beauty of your experience. You can also reduce worry, nervousness, and bad feelings that might interfere with your pleasure.

You can practice mindfulness in any setting, but here are some guided mini-mindfulness routines that you can apply to some common activities: Eating a piece of fruit: Before you eat, notice the color, shape, and feel of the fruit. Bring it to your nose and smell its aroma. Take a bite and notice the taste, sweetness, and juiciness. Chew slowly and enjoy each bite. Pay

Long-Term Success: Staying Quit, Forever

You've made it through the first few weeks of stopping smoking. Congratulations! You've passed the most tough part of the process, and you should be proud of yourself. You've also started to rewire your reward system by finding new joys in life and practicing awareness.

But stopping smoking is not a one-time thing. It's a lifelong journey, and it's not always a straight line. There may be days when you feel tempted to smoke again, or when you face stressful events that test your determination. That's okay. It's normal to have ups and downs, and it doesn't mean you've failed.

In this section, we will show you how to stay quiet, forever. You will learn how to build your relapse prevention tools, a set of techniques that can help you cope with any cravings or triggers that might arise. You will also learn how to keep your smoke-free lifestyle, by building an ongoing practice that supports your well-being. Finally, you will find the ripple effect of your choice to quit, and how it can inspire others to follow your example.

Building Your Relapse Prevention Toolkit

Even after you've quit smoking, you may still face scenarios that spark your desire to smoke. These could be external factors, such as people, places, or events that remind you of smoking. Or they could be internal factors, such as feelings, thoughts, or experiences that make you crave a cigarette.

The key to avoiding relapse is to spot these triggers and apply your tools to deal with them. Here are some examples of how you can do that:

- Recognize the trigger: Identify what is making you want to smoke. Is it a person, a place, a feeling, or something else? Be detailed and honest with yourself.
- Deploy your tools: Use one or more of the techniques that you've learned to deal with the cause. For example, you can:
- Take a few deep breaths and rest your body and mind.

- Distract yourself with a different task, such as reading, playing a game, or calling a friend.
- Remind yourself of your reasons for stopping, and the benefits you've gained.
- Reach out to a support person, such as a family member, a friend, or a psychologist, and talk to them about how you feel. Use a nicotine replacement product, such as a patch, a gum, or a lozenge, if you need extra help.
- Analyze and learn: If you manage to fight the urge to smoke, praise yourself and reward yourself with something healthy and enjoyable. If you slip and smoke, don't beat yourself up or give up. Instead, try to learn from the event, and think about what you can do better next time.

Maintenance Mode

After a few months of stopping smoking, you may notice that your cravings become less regular and strong. You may also feel more confident and comfortable in your smoke-free life. This is a great sign that you've made a permanent change.

But don't let your guard down. Even after years of being smoke-free, you may still face settings that tempt you to smoke again. For example, you may meet a former smoking buddy, or go through a big life change, such as a divorce, a loss, or a retirement.

That's why it's important to keep your smoke-free lifestyle in upkeep mode. This means that you continue to watch your thoughts and behaviors and take steps to avoid relapse. Here are some ideas for building an ongoing "staying quiet" practice:

Monthly check-ins:

Once a month, take some time to analyze how you feel about being smoke-free. Ask yourself things such as:

- How often do I think about smoking?
- How do I deal with urges or triggers?
- What are the perks of being smoke-free?
- What are the difficulties of being smoke-free?
- What are my plans for the next month?

Occasional support: Even if you don't need daily or weekly support, it can still be helpful to seek occasional support from others who understand what

My Reward System Worksheet

Instructions:

- **Rediscover What Brings You Joy:** Take some time to reflect on things you already appreciate. Sometimes, smoking has overshadowed these basic delights.

- **Explore New Possibilities:** Think about activities you've always wanted to try or used to adore but haven't done in a while.

- **Rate and Categorize:** Use the space below to organize your rewards and assign them a "Joy Rating". The categories are suggestions – feel free to construct your own!

My Existing Pleasures

Relaxing Rewards: (Things that help you decompress and de-stress)

Example: Taking a warm bath, reading a nice book, listening to tranquil music.

Your Ideas: ______________Joy Rating (1-5): _______

Creative Rewards: (Things that express your creativity or inspire inquiry)

Example: Drawing/painting, playing an instrument, attempting a novel recipe

Your Ideas: ______________ Joy Rating (1-5): _______

Active Rewards: (Things that get you moving and feeling wonderful)

Example: Going for a walk, dancing, extending

Your Ideas: ______________Joy Rating (1-5): _______

Social Rewards: (Things that involve connecting with others)

Example: Catching up with an acquaintance, spending time with family, joining a club

Your Ideas:______________ Joy Rating (1-5): _______

Rewards I Want to Explore

Brainstorm at least 3-5 new things you'd like to attempt.
Big or minor, let your curiosity guide you!

Next Steps

- Circle 1-2 "Existing Pleasures" to savor mindfully throughout the week.
- Pick ONE "Reward to Explore" and take action to make it happen this week!
- Notes and Reflections: Use this space to monitor how these rewards make you feel, and any surprises, or obstacles you encounter.

Additional Tips:

- Small and Accessible: Focus on rewards easily implemented into ordinary life.
- Visualize: Add a section for drawing or pasting images of rewards for extra inspiration

- Revisit and Update: This is an ongoing tool to refine as you progress on your smoke-free voyage.

My Cravings Action Plan

Instructions:

- Know Your Triggers: Think about the most prevalent situations, emotions, or times of day that make you desire a cigarette. List your top 3-5 triggers below.

- Build Your Toolbox: For EACH trigger, choose 2-3 strategies from the suggestions below, or come up with your own ideas. The key is to have multiple options available to deploy.

- Escalation Plan: If your customary go-to tactics fail and the craving intensifies, what's your next move? It might be reaching out for support or having an "emergency" distraction technique.

My Triggers and Action Steps:

My Top Triggers:

Trigger   1:

____

Action Step A: _______________________________________
Action Step B: _______________________________________
Action Step C: _______________________________________

Trigger   2:

____

Action Step A: _______________________________________
Action Step B: _______________________________________
Action Step C: _______________________________________

[Repeat format for 3-5 triggers]

My Escalation Plan (When Cravings Get Intense):

Craving Combat Toolbox (Suggestions)

- Deep Breathing: Focus on slow, controlled abdominal breathing.
- Mindful Movement: A few minutes of stretching, strolling, or uncomplicated exercise.
- Sensory Shift: Smell something pungent (essential oil), chew sugar-free gum, and bite on a hard confectionery.
- Engage Your Mind: Do a puzzle, read an absorbing article, or play a game on your phone.
- Reach Out: Text a support person, or visit an online cessation forum.
- Step Away: Physically alter your environment – go outside, take a shower, etc.
- Important Notes:
- Practice Makes Perfect: Visualize using this plan when you're not yearning.
- No Shame: If you give in, analyze why and modify your plan, don't tear yourself up.

- Seek Help: If cravings feel overwhelming, contact a therapist or addiction support hotline.

Quitting smoking isn't just about deprivation; it's an opportunity to rewire your brain for greater pleasure and fulfillment in ways you might not have envisaged while under nicotine's control.

Conclusion: Your Smoke-Free Future Begins Now

Look at how far you've come! You've faced the grip of smoking head-on and emerged on the other side. Whether you're a day, a week, or many months into this journey, you've opened a strength within you that many never find.

The road ahead won't always be perfectly smooth. There may be times when old urges flicker, or worry feels overwhelming. Remember, these are temporary tests of your willpower, and each task you beat makes you even stronger.

You now have the tools, the information, and the unwavering belief in yourself to handle whatever comes your way. You know the science behind addiction, you've mastered your breath and honed the power of your mind. But most importantly, you've reconnected with the core reason why you picked this route.

Imagine your smoke-free future stretching ahead of you. Days filled with energy, nights filled with peaceful sleep, and years filled with things you wouldn't trade for any cigarette. Imagine the joy shining in the eyes of your loved ones, and the great example you set for those around you.

This isn't just about stopping; it's about change. It's about recovering your freedom, your health, and the very best version of yourself. You may have started this book as a smoker, but you finish it as someone who defeated addiction.

And if there's one thing we know for sure, it's this: You've got this.

Author's message

If you're reading this, you're ready for a change. You've probably tried to quit before and I know how challenging it can be. I wrote this book because I believe most traditional methods fail smokers, setting them up for frustration. I want you to know that lasting freedom from nicotine is possible. This book is your roadmap, providing the tools, knowledge, and unwavering support to guide you every step of the way.